Water Fasting

Rapid Weight Loss, Revitalized Health and Body Cleansing Through Water Fasting

Michael D Kaiser

Water Fasting: Rapid Weight Loss, Revitalized Health and Body Cleansing Through Water Fasting

Published by:
Dana Publishing Inc., 12804 Chillicothe Road #202
Chesterland, Ohio 44026, United States of America
Cover art by Dana Onyshko

Table of Contents

Introduction

What is your goal right?

- Lose weight?
- Improve your health?
- Lower your blood pressure?
- Feel less bloated, increase metabolism and cell repair?

Did you know that water fasting is the answer to all of the above?

While fasting is a concept that has been around for thousands of years, water fasting is a concept that is relatively new. It may seem like an almost impossible concept to think that the human body can survive for a prolonged period on nothing but water—but when performed carefully, it is entirely possible, as you are about to discover during the next few chapters of this book.

Back in ancient times, a fast was a mandatory practice before men went to war. It was also a coming-of-age ritual that was practiced when a woman or man came of age. In other cultures, fasting was used to assuage angry deities and to avoid catastrophes such as flood and famine.

Fasting has evolved since then and today is primarily regaining its popularity because of the numerous benefits associated with this practice. You are now about to embark on a journey towards better health in a way that doesn't involve quick fixes or unhealthy weight loss supplements. You are about to embark on a life-changing health journey that requires you to do nothing more than to abstain from food for a certain period of time.

Chapter 1: Fasting and the Human Body

Understanding the science of water fasting is crucial to doing it right. You do not want to go about doing a fast without knowing the how-to's and even the why's. Thus, let's start off with a little bit of history.

History of Fasting

Many of the first advocates of fasting were from Greece, particularly Pythagoras, who extolled its many virtues. St. Catherine of Siena practiced fasting in the fourteenth century, while Doctor Paracelsus called it the "physician within" in the Renaissance period.

Fasting in its various forms is a distinguished tradition and one that runs throughout centuries with devotees claiming spiritual and physical renewal of body, mind, and spirit.

Back in ancient times, a fast was a mandatory practice before men went to war. It was also a coming-of-age ritual that was practiced when a woman or man came of age. In other cultures, fasting was used to assuage angry deities and to avoid catastrophes such as flood and famine.

In many of the world's major religions, fasting plays a key role in its practice, and it is associated with forms of self-control as well as penitence.

For example, in Judaism, they usually go through an annual fast called Yom Kippur, which is the Day of Atonement. In Islam, the holy month of Ramadan is when a fast from sunrise to sunset is observed.

In Roman Catholicism, as well as in the Eastern Orthodox, a 40-day fast is observed during Lent just as how Christ fasted in the desert for 40 days. For some reason, women seem to be major proponents of religious fasting, as it was seen as a sign of chastity as well as holiness.

The English anchoress and mystic known as Julian of Norwich, who lived around the 14th century, fasted for lengthy periods of time because she saw it as a means of communication with Christ. In other systems of beliefs, it was thought that Gods revealed their divine teachings and visions through dreams of temple priests.

Fasting is also used as a gesture of political protest. The most classic example of this is through the Suffragettes movement as well as Mahatma Gandhi, who went through 17 fasting sessions as a sign of protest to the British rule and for the struggle of India's independence.

While fasting done right is good, some have taken on an excessive concept of fasting. Take, for example, the case of Dr. Linda Burfield Hazzard, who caused the death of over 40 of her patients whom she instructed to go on an extreme fast. This doctor from Minnesota was eventually convicted of manslaughter back in 1912. In 1938, she died of her own strict regime of fasting.

There were also the Victorian fasting girls whose claims were that they could sustain without food. Then there was the doctor of the Art of Natural Hygiene Movement, Dr. Herbert Shelton who has claimed to have helped over 40,000 people with their health problems.

Across the pond in the UK, fasting was considered as part of the 'Nature Cure' movement that stressed the importance of sunshine, fresh air, exercise as well as 'positive thinking' to cure oneself of health-related problems. Fasting was extremely popular in the 1920s, and the first Nature Cure clinic opened up in Edinburgh. From then on, other clinics focusing on therapeutic fasting started blooming such as the legendary known Tyringham Hall located in Buckinghamshire as well as Champneys located in Hertfordshire. While it was initially deemed as a naturopathic center, it is now known as a destination spa in the modern world.

Fasting was known to cure many a disease such as those related to heart, obesity, high blood pressure, allergies, and digestive issues as well as headaches. These fasting sessions were tailored to meet the individuals' specific needs, and it could be a fast that is just for a day or two or can go up to 2 to three months. These clinics would take into account the individual's full medical history to see if they were able to go through a fast or not—and if they were suitable, these patients would be monitored closely.

As the years went by and medical technology kept evolving and becoming better, the natural cure of ailments fell out of favor by the British and was soon replaced by better drugs and more advanced health care methods.

In Germany, by contrast, fasting was gaining ground especially through the pioneering works of Dr. Otto Buchinger. German hospitals also run fasting weeks as part of a complementing treatment to help manage different kinds of diseases such as obesity and blood pressure.

In other parts of Europe such as Hungary, Czech Republic, and Austria, centers and spas are quite popular, which offer fasting holidays. Fasting in Germany is referred to as "naturheilkunde," which means natural health practice. It is still extremely popular in the country because it has been integrated into modern medical practices, which means these fasts can be administered by doctors to their patients.

In the US, fasting has been increasingly growing as millions of people try on fasts such as Intermittent Fasting and Water Fasting to maintain their health and weight. This renewed interest is welcomed by the medical community, as it helps mitigate the toxic effects of daily living and gives the body a "break."

What Is Water Fasting?

Now that have a little bit of history to fasting, let's talk a little deeper about Water Fasting. Essentially, water fasting is just another type of fast that only allows you to consume water. These fasts usually can be between 24 hours to 72 hours. During this time, a person does not consume any kinds of food and only consumes water.

It is strongly advised not to fast any longer than the period of 24 to 72 hours unless you have medical clearance and under supervision.

Why would anyone want to fast for that long? There are plenty of reasons why a person would go fasting by only consuming water. These reasons are:

- For religious purposes
- For spiritual reasons
- To detox the body of toxins
- For the health benefits of fasting
- To prepare for a medical procedure or operation

Plenty of people undertake water fast for its health benefits, and it is also because there are plenty of benefits related to a water fast such as lowering the risk of cancer, diabetes as well as heart diseases.

Water fasting has been known to promote a process called autophagy where the body can break down and recycle parts of the cells that may be dangerous. Diets such as the lemon detox have been fashioned after the water fast. The lemon detox fast allows you to drink, for several times a day, a mixture of water, lemon juice with a little bit of cayenne pepper or maple syrup added into it for up to seven days.

Where water fasting is concerned, while it does have its health benefits, it is not something without its risks, and it can be dangerous if the fast is prolonged.

What Happens in the 24 to 72 Hours of a Water Fast?

During a water fast, you can only drink water and not consume any kind of food or even beverage such as juices. You need to drink at least two to three liters of water each day, between 24 to 72 hours.

Never, ever go beyond this point of time to fast without medical supervision. Confining yourself to an all-water diet for more than 72 hours is hazardous to your health, doing more harm than good.

While in water fasting, it is easy to feel dizzy or weak especially if you are new to this. During this time, low-intensity work is best, so avoid operating heavy machinery, rigorous exercise or even high-intensity workouts.

What Happens to Your Body When You Fast?

The first few hours into the fast are pretty normal. People usually can last without feeling dizzy or weak. This is because your body is going through its regular process of storing glucose and breaking down glycogen. In most circumstances, 25% of glucose goes directly to the brain whereas the rest is used to support your muscles and blood cells.

After about five to six hours, most people reach a state of ketosis. This depends on your body's sugar levels- some people take faster, and some people take a slower time to reach ketosis. Ketosis is the metabolic state of the body where energy levels are supported by ketones in your blood. This is the process of breaking down fat. This is when the real fasting begins, and it is the most desirable state to be in for people fasting to lose weight. This state can also be reached through a ketogenic diet which is a low-carb, high-fat diet.

When your body goes into ketosis, other things tend to happen such as the release of cholesterol as well as uric acid into the bloodstream. This is an essential process because it detoxifies the body.

At this state, most people start experiencing dizziness, headaches, skin rashes even as well as fatigue. The lesser known symptoms are that of muscle pain and joint aches. At the ending of this stage, the pain begins to lessen, and the blood pressure will drop. This process is called calcification process where the mucoid plaque, as well as the cholesterol in the body, will reduce.

When our food intake has been reduced, this gives our digestive system a rest. However, since the process of digestion takes a little time, it is never fully stopped when we fast intermittently. The digestive process only fully rests when we go through a more prolonged fast.

After the first 6 hours of fasting, you will end up feeling hungry, naturally and also slightly overwhelmed. This could trigger certain emotional states such as frustration, anger, sadness and even feeling depressed.

If you are fasting for an extended period, allow yourself to deal with these emotions as they come and also to keep telling yourself that the way you feel is happening due to the fast you are undergoing.

You do not want to take out your emotions on the people around you—which is why fasting also should come with meditation. This helps because it takes your mind away from the hunger and instead focuses it on activities that you can do without much bodily effort.

Chapter 2: Processes Involving Water Fasting

The Stages of Water Fasting

Stage 1

The first stage usually starts from the time you take your last meal and lasts up to about 12-48 hours. Before embarking on this type of fast, it is always recommended to undergo proper planning way ahead of time to ensure the successful completion of the fasting period.

The first stage is typically the most challenging stage that you would have to go through at the beginning of the fast. At this stage, you will begin to feel hunger pangs due to your normal meal cycles as your body starts to adjust itself during this fasting phase. It is also not uncommon to feel low in energy or end up in negative mood swings during this period.

The feeling of 'low energy" occurs when the body starts to adapt during this fasting period when it starts to use less energy. This includes lowering your blood pressure and your heart rate. This process is called "gluconeogenesis," and it is a process where the liver starts to convert fats and amino acids into glucose to obtain the energy it needs for proper bodily functions.

Stage 2

Stage two begins after the first forty-eight hours and will last right up to the seventh day. At this phase, changes in your physical appearance will start to occur, and you are entering what is known as "ketosis." At this stage, the body will start to convert the fat stored in your body as fuel. Hence, you might stop feeling moody and hungry during this period.

Stage 3

Stage three will take place from days eight to fifteen, and you will start to experience changes to your mood. At this stage, your body becomes fully adjusted to the "fasting" stage, and your digestive systems go into a "relaxation" phase. Since you haven't been consuming any solid food or liquids for the better part of the last ten days, the body and digestive system have lesser work to do in breaking downs foods into the bloodstream. When you have entered this phase, you will notice an improvement to your overall wellbeing and increased energy levels plus an improved clarity of mind.

Stage 4

Day sixteen and beyond is when you have entered stage four of the fasting experience. This will then continue on towards the end of the fasting period. We advise that if you do reach this stage, you should consult your doctor and ensure the continuation of this stage is done under your doctor's supervision. Stage four of the fasting process is the culmination of the repairing and cleansing process of your body that began with the earlier stages. As such, the longer you fast, the more time the body has the chance to heal itself.

Stage 5

When to break a fast is subjective, and it depends totally up to you and your goals. It is important that when you choose to break your fast, you should take your time to re-adjust to consuming solid foods. Your body and digestive system need time to re-configure back into its normal routine after such a long period of an extended fast. It's best that you ease your way back into this by consuming soups and vegetables as a start. Also consuming fruit juices will also help accomplish the fast-breaking phase.

Ways to Prepare Your Body

Planning is a key component in the successful completion of water fast. Therefore, it is imperative that you should begin preparing your body and mind in the best way possible during this period. First and foremost, it is ultimately important to seek medical consultation from your doctor before getting into this type of fast. Should you not be in the best shape, the risks that can occur will far outweigh the benefits that can be derived from fasting. Also, those experiencing any medical conditions such as low blood pressure, diabetes, those who are underweight and women in pregnancy should avoid fasting. As such, a proper medical examination to clear yourself as fit before undertaking this type of fast is critical.

The fasting period will cause a lot of changes to your mental state as well. Since you will be experiencing bouts of hunger during the initial stages of the fast, it is also important to prepare mentally for the challenge ahead. So, it is important to ease yourself during the initial stages by being aware and controlling your hunger pangs and mood swings that can occur due to low energy levels. You may also be affected by diarrhea, headaches, fatigue, and body odor due to the elimination of waste and toxins in your body. To accommodate these effects, you could opt to take some time off work to put yourself in a relaxed environment and ease your way into the entire fasting process.

You should start this process slowly by "detoxifying" your body. Begin by eliminating foods such as meats, eggs, fish, milk, and cheese. Stop drinking coffee, sugary drinks, and even alcohol. If you are a smoker, best to gradually reduce your smoking habits and coming to a complete stop just before your fasting period is scheduled to begin. Alter your habits of eating by consuming rawer and more wholesome foods such as vegetables, fruits, and grains—and slowly start to consume less and less food as you head towards your fasting deadline.

You may also prepare your body a few weeks ahead before your water fast by utilizing the intermittent fasting method to get your body prepared and train yourself to control your hunger pangs. A simple four-week plan would be as follows:

Week 1: Skip eating breakfast.

Week 2: Skip both breakfast and lunch.

Week 3: Skip all three meals and control your portions for dinner.

Week 4: Water Fast begins!

In the week or days leading up to the start of your fast, you will need to increase your water intake to prepare your body for a fast period and to ensure it is well-hydrated. Lastly, ensure that you get enough sleep and rest before and during your fasting period to ensure your body is fully rested and recovered pre and during your fasting window.

How Long You Should Fast

The standard fasting period can vary between one to forty days based on the type of goal that you are planning on achieving. For any fasts that last up to forty days, you will need to get your doctor's approval before doing so. Below is a simple guideline, from Dr. David Jockers, a doctor of natural medicine on the duration and frequency of fasting based on your overall goals.

For thin or lean individuals who are looking to reduce inflammation and chronic diseases, you should typically strive for a fast between three to five days and repeat this process every two to three months.

For individuals within your normal BMI weight rating, who also are looking to reduce inflammation and chronic diseases, you should target for a fast that's between four to seven days and repeat this process for each one and a half to two months. For individuals that are considered overweight, who are not only looking to reduce inflammation and chronic diseases but also aiming to shed their excess weight, they should target a longer fast period that's between five to ten (or more) days and repeat this process every month.

It is important to note that even if you are in the pink of health, undergoing extended periods of water fasting can help battle diseases and help regulate optimal body weight and composition.

Tips for Taking Care of Yourself When You Fast

Experiencing low levels of energy during the early stage of the fasting period are common, and it will be important that you get plenty of rest during this period. Ensure that you maintain an interrupted sleep cycle with a minimum of seven to eight hours of sleep per day. If you need a short power nap during the day, take it. Never overexert yourself during this period. As such, you may also want to prevent for indulging in any cardio or weightlifting exercises during this period as it may only crank up your hunger levels. Try low impact activities such as stretching and yoga during the period you are practicing this fast. It will also be helpful to undergo a massage session that can make the fasting process more enjoyable and help with the detoxification of the body.

Keep yourself hydrated. Try to aim between nine to thirteen glasses of water per day during your fast period. Drink only pure water, or you may also opt for distilled water. It is also recommended that if you should feel dizzy, take a pinch of salt and drink it with 250 ml of water. This should balance back your insulin levels in the body. Periodically drinking the water will also help to combat the hunger pangs that you will feel especially within the first few days of the fast. It is also important to note that, try to breakdown the consumption of water equally throughout the entire day. Don't drink it all at once.

Dizziness is also a common symptom that is experienced by those undergoing prolonged periods of fasting. This usually occurs when you get up too fast. Practice getting up slowly to avoid the sudden blood rush to the head. Some deep breathing will also help negate this effect. Try to sit or lie down when you get dizzy. Rest until it passes. If symptoms persist and get worst, stop your fasting and immediately consult a doctor on your condition. Bare feet walking outside on grass or dirt can also be very helpful during this stage. By enabling your body's own electromagnetic current to ground itself into the Earth, you will be allowing the healthy electromagnetic frequencies from the Earth run through you and act as a form of antioxidants.

If you find yourself in a colder climate, you may opt to do this using a pair of socks instead of going barefoot. This method helps to improve your mental clarity and aid in relaxation during the fasting period. Keeping a log during your fasting journey may also help you mentally in the successful completion of the fast. Keeping notes each day of your body changes, how you feel, and what you eat can keep you focused on the journey and ensure you stay on track.

Other smaller action items that you can practice during this period are: -

- Using a dry brush when showering (two to four times a day) to enable the skin to expel toxins. Also advisable to bath in warm water to open up the pores of the skin.
- Use activated charcoal powder to brush your teeth and tongue as bad breath is common when fasting for prolonged periods.
- Ensure proper ventilation in any room that you are in as body odor is also an issue when fasting.

Chapter 3: Water Fast How-To

How Long Should You Water Fast for?

When it comes to water fasting, this is the most searched-for answer. The optimum fast is three days, which fit well for a weekend fast. However, there are other standard lengths that you may consider. Whatever the length you choose, you must give careful consideration, and you must speak to your doctor about it before attempting this type of fast or any other kind of fast.

If you have never tried to fast before, then committing for a few hours a day would help you familiarize yourself with the sensations and the process. Your first fast should give you an idea of how your body can handle itself while fasting. You need to learn about your body by going through this on your own because everybody is unique.

Transition Periods

You need to keep in mind that the actual fast is much shorter than the time commitment to get your body to the state of fasting. This is usually called transition periods both occurring before and after the fast where you wash your way out of a full diet and then again, easing back to normal eating.

This transition period can be based on the length of the fast itself. You need to take half the number of days for the fast for your transition period. What you are doing here is to double the number of days from start to finish. For example, if your fast is for 10 days, then you need to commit to a total of 20 days of attention. A three day fast would essentially take 6 days of attention and commitment.

For most people, they feel 4 days is sufficient enough for transitioning before and after a lengthy fast. This is, of course, depending on your post-fast goals- will you stick to a healthier eating plan or will you be going back to a binge junk-food eating spree?

If you are attempting a three-day fast period, you want to allocate at least a day before and after for transitioning. Consider how a warm-up exercise and cool-down exercise benefits the body? The transitioning period also works the same way.

For instance, a three day fast would require a day before and after the fast. Keep in mind that the longer you take to acclimate your body prior to the fast, the easier your fast will become.

You can start by scaling back on your meal portions or even just opting to fast for more hours each day.

Choosing a Length

So what is a good length of time to fast for you?

Your chosen length of time for fasting must always be the right length for you at the time you are considering it. You must not be rigid and be flexible in your fast because things could happen to your body which would require you to end the fast and begin eating immediately, such as getting a cold or even a stomachache. You can back off a bit if you feel any discomfort and eat a little bit of fresh fruit.

You must also have a goal in mind before you begin your fast so that you can be adequately prepared for it. You must also not attempt to do this too frequently. Your body needs sufficient time to rebuild its nutritional reserves after a fast.

The recommended fasting times for body maintenance and balancing is one day per week or 3 days per month or 10 days a year.

Most Common Lengths for Fasting

- One week fast – this is often done as a quarterly cleansing detox.

- 10-day fast – among the popular options of fasting, this is the standard fasting time recommended in the Master

Cleanse detox diet. Plenty of people use this 10-day fast as a yearly detox and cleansing mechanism.

Essentially, the length of time for your fast depends also on the goals you want to accomplish:

1. Three-day water fast - helps in getting rid of toxins and cleanses the blood
2. Five-day fast - renews and heals the body's immune system
3. Ten-day fast - prevents future problems with the body and prevents illnesses such as a degenerative disease

Beginning Your Fast — Starting with a Supervised Fast

In the documentary created in 2016 called 'The Science of Fasting,' it covers issues and studies related to penguins that fasted for three to four months at a time. The documentary also covered the effects of fasting on rats done by researchers in California. While the documentary could be dry, it can help you in finding out more about the benefits and effects of fasting.

When you begin your water fast, you want to consider doing a supervised fast, especially if your goals are to alleviate serious diseases and conditions.

Water fasting can be dangerous, and it is extremely important to note that you should only do it for a maximum of 72 hours. The most common and serious problem related to water fasting is sustaining an injury from passing out.

With a supervised fast, you can get tests done before you start fasting to ensure that you do not have any physical issues or concerns that may complicate the fast.

Supervised fasting is also good especially for those who are overweight, and they want to lose weight fast. Obesity itself presents its own set of challenges, and most people already have some form of addiction or severe eating pattern.

Another reason for getting your fast supervised is to ensure that you do not have emotional attachments with your food. You must be careful not to support a behavior that could potentially lead to an eating disorder. Instead, fasting must be with the end goal to promote a healthier lifestyle and better eating habits.

How to Find Someone to Supervise Your Water Fast

You may not have any particular health issues that may complicate the fast, but it never hurts to get your fast supervised especially if this is your first time doing it.

You could have a medical expert help you with the fast by going through the length of time, speaking to you about any concerns and uncertainties as well as checking up on you while you are undergoing the fast.

Experts who frequently supervise fasts are familiar with the changes that the body goes through and how they respond during the fasting period would be able to offer you practices that are best suited to your needs. They would also be able to advise you if fasting is something not worth doing for your body.

Most experts will require you to go to their clinics or retreat centers, but there are also a few that offer their services via YouTube or Skype so you can fast in the comforts of your own home. If you have a certain medical condition, then you would be advised by fasting experts or supervisors to visit your local doctor regularly to check if your vitals are in good balance.

If you cannot find a suitable fasting supervisor, clinics, or retreats in your area, then another good option is to talk to your doctor that you see frequently and check to see if they could oversee your health while you are doing a water fast.

However, medical doctors are not really familiar with fasting and may even recommend that you do not do it.

Going at It Alone

While having an expert by your side is beneficial in water fasting, many people have attempted it successfully on their own. Usually, in these scenarios, a rational mind and intuitive knowledge of your own body are sufficient enough to help you know when a fast is too much and keep you out of danger. Do not bite more than you can chew, so if this is your first time, do not attempt 3-day water fast immediately. Start with a short, one-day fast that is easier, or go through intermittent fasting and break your fast with light food such as juices or fresh fruits.

You may also want to kick-off a cleansing diet a week or two prior to your water fast, especially if you already have poor eating habits. This will help eliminate as many toxins before the actual water fast and not make your body too overwhelmed.

Gaining some experience from your fast such as how your body reacts, the emotional triggers you may have during your fast are all helpful in gathering the knowledge about your body and what it takes to fast.

You may also realize that three-day water fast is not for you, and you may just end up sticking to once a week water fasts. These shorter bursts of fasts can be informative to you, and it can clarify your relationship with food, making it better.

Fasting, in its many forms, is an amazing personal gift to ourselves. If you have no desire to stick to long-term fasts, then sticking to short term fasts will help your body over time. If you are going to do a water fast on your own, then you must honor the rules of fasting which are resting and recuperating.

You must slow down and honor the needs of your body and the messages it is sending you. Fasting is about healing on all levels- mentally, physically as well as emotionally and only you know what needs to be done.

Water fasting is no joke so keep an open mind and be flexible. Read as much as you can do know the benefits, side effects and other elements that come into play when you water fast.

Remember that you are not competing with anyone. This is your body so only fast for as long as you can and for as long as it is recommended to be safe.

Listening to your own inner guidance and signals are essential when you fast and do not succumb to the pressure that other people are watching you.

Tips of Sustaining Yourself During the Fast

Here are some quick tips in helping you sustain a healthy and safe fast:

1. Keep Fasting Periods Short

If this is your first time fasting, keep it short. Remember that there is no one you are competing with. Start with shorter fast periods before going into a full day fast.

2. Eat a Small Amount on Fast Days

If you feel like you are doing to faint and drinking water alone is not helping, then eat small amounts of food to sustain you on your fast days. It will do more good than harm.

3. Stay Hydrated

Of course, water fast needs water. Keep drinking water as often and as much as you can. If you ever feel like you need some electrolytes, squeeze in some lemon juice to your bottle of water.

4. Meditate

Meditation helps the mind and body focus and be one. Meditation also helps you keep your thoughts away from food and cravings. A 10-minute meditation every morning can help center yourself as well as keep your awareness in your mind and focused on your fasting goals.

5. Don't Break Fasts with a Feast

When it is time to break your fast, don't go in with a large amount of food. Start small such as with a piece of fruit, a glass of milk or even fruit juice helps. This prevents the body from going into a shock.

6. Stop Fasting If You Feel Unwell

When you feel like you cannot sustain any longer, you keep feeling dizzy, you start coughing or feel like a fever is coming, then stop. There is no point fasting if you are feeling unwell.

7. Eat Plenty of Whole Foods on Non-Fasting Days

A good way to sustain future fasting periods is to eat whole foods because eating balanced and wholesome meals help curb cravings towards sugar and carbs and help you develop a more sophisticated palate.

8. Keep Exercise Mild

You can choose to exercise if you want during your fast, but if you do, then you must keep it mild. Yoga, meditation, stretching, and a little bit of brisk walking helps.

Chapter 4: Advantages of a Water Fast and Its Weight Loss Benefits

While fasting is a concept that has been around for thousands of years, water fasting is a concept that is relatively new. It may seem like an almost impossible concept to think that the human body can survive for a prolonged period on nothing but water, but when performed carefully, it is entirely possible. Not only that—there are several advantages and benefits, which include weight loss, that you could gain from it as well.

Needless to say, fasting has existed for as long as it did because of the numerous benefits associated with this practice. With water fasting, you're restricting your intake to everything *except* water. Water is literally the only thing that your body is allowed to consume while you're undergoing the process. Whether it's 24 hours or 72 hours, during the hours that you've committed to your water fast, your body is not going to see anything else except a continuous intake of water.

Water is the life force of all things on earth. Including the human body. 60% of our bodies comprise of water, and it is this very crucial, vital element that helps keeps us alive. Water flows throughout the cells in our bodies, our tissues, and our organs, helping us to maintain our bodily functions as we go about your day. We need water in order to survive. Besides helping with all these bodily functions, water also helps us maintain a healthy digestive system. Now, if we're already drinking water on a daily basis, why do we need to perform water fast specifically?

Why has this method become so popular recently? Because of the advantages that are touted with this approach and the weight loss benefits associated with it. While some amount of weight loss is experienced with almost any fasting method which is done consistently, water fasting is about more than just weight loss. It's about *overall health.*

Advantages of Water Fasting

If you're thinking about starting the water fasting method for your personal health reasons, you'll be pleased to find that you are likely to experience the following advantages:

It Potentially Helps with Autophagy Promotion. *Healthline.com,* an online health & wellness publication, revealed that several studies had discovered water fasting may help with the promotion of autophagy in your body. Autophagy is what happens when older parts of the cells in your body get broken down and then recycled, which could potentially help to protect you against certain illnesses such as heart disease, cancer or Alzheimer's for example. Autophagy could potentially prevent the damaged cells from accumulating unhealthily in your body, which then minimizes the risk factors which are associated with cancer and minimize the chances of cancer cells growing. However, there is still not enough study conducted on just how effective water fasting is in terms of autophagy promotion, and more research into the field is needed.

It Could Potentially Help to Lower Your Blood Pressure. A study which was published by NCBI indicated that after research, prolonged water fasts which are performed under medical supervision could help those who are suffering from high blood pressure. That same study revealed that 68 individuals who were dealing with borderline high blood pressure were put under medical supervision as they underwent water fasting for a period of 14-days (almost). By the time they reached the end of their fasting period, the results had revealed that 82% of those individuals witnessed a significant difference in their blood pressure levels, which had now dropped to considerably healthier levels. Another study involved a group of 174 individuals who were dealing with high blood pressure and saw them undergo the water fasting method for an average period of 10 and 11 days. By the end of that period, 90% of those surveyed saw a drop in their blood pressure to 140/90mmHg. There have not been enough studies conducted on whether this same result can be achieved with short-term water fasts and blood pressure (where fasts range anywhere from 24 to 72 hours).

It Could Potentially Improve Sensitivity to Leptin and Insulin. The human body's metabolism is affected by two very important hormones, known as leptin and insulin. Once again, NCBI revealed research water fasting could potentially lead the body towards becoming more sensitive towards insulin and leptin, which means these hormones become a lot more effective. Improved insulin sensitivity means that the body will be more efficient in the reduction of blood sugar, while improved leptin sensitivity helps your body deal and process with hunger signals. Managing your hunger signals effectively, in turn, will reduce the risk of experiencing obesity.

It Could Help to Reduce Inflammation in Your Body. According to research which was conducted by the Yale School of Medicine, discovered that fasting could help to minimize inflammation and pro-inflammatory cytokines in the human body. It could also help to lower the oxidative damage happening within the body. The researches at Yale School discovered that the hydroxybutyrate (BHB) compound inhibits NLRP3, which is one part of a set of proteins known as inflammasome. This is responsible for the inflammatory response that the body gives out in several diseases, which include autoimmune disease, Alzheimer's, heart disease and even Type 2 diabetes. What these researchers found was that BHB was best produced through fasting, which was by far the most effective method. Other methods include exercises performed at high intensity, the ketogenic diet, and a restriction in calorie intake.

It Could Help to Boost Your Body's Immune System. A University of California Professor of Gerontology and Biological Sciences, Dr. Valter Longo, in a study conducted in 2014 discovered that 3-day water fast could help the body regenerate its immune system. Fasting helped the body turn on its regenerative switch, which then prompted stem cells to go into their regenerative mode and produce new white blood cells. Fasting, according to Dr. Longo, tells the body that it is OK to go ahead with the proliferation process and rebuild its system. A study by the University of California Berkeley also backed that up with research that revealed a 3-day water fast was what the body exactly needed to help reset its immune system, helping you then to perform at your most optimum level.

It Allows Your Body to Reset. It's no secret that our bodies are exposed to unhealthier food options and lifestyle choices these days. Fast food, processed foods, fatty foods, you name it, we've all consumed it at some point or other. Some people may even consume it more than they should because of their hectic, on-the-go lifestyles—which is why it is crucial for us to help our bodies reset every once in a while, and the water fast is one of the best methods to do that. Water is the only thing that is 100% good for the human body with no adverse side effects, the way a lot of other foods and liquids might have.

Weight Loss Benefits of Water Fasting

Now, this is the big question that those who are keen on losing weight will be curious to know: *does water fasting help with weight loss?*

It will, but there is a difference between losing weight and *burning fat.* Water fasting is not going to help you with the latter—which means that the majority of your weight loss is going to be a result of your body losing water, muscle mass during the fast and carbs. Not so much about fat burning. In general, it takes several days for the human body to start using their fat stores as fuel, so if you're after a fast fat burning fasting method, another approach may suit you better.

Of course, that's not to say that no weight loss is going to happen. There will be some amount of weight loss benefits that you'll experience with the water fast, especially if you do it consistently. Everyone's bodies work differently—some experience a greater level of weight loss than others. With the water-fast method, the first initial stages are going to involve a loss in water weight, and the fat burning only kicks it at a later stage when your body has been deprived of food long enough.

Toronto-based acupuncturist and chiropractor, Ben Kim, mentions that at least one pound a day of weight loss can be expected when undergoing the water fast (again, not everyone's bodies are going to work the same way). Some people may even lose as much as 3 pounds a day, especially if you've previously consumed a diet which involves a large number of processed foods where a lot of water has been retained.

Whether we like it or not, there is no one, sure-fire approach method to weight loss. Water fasting, while highly beneficial for your body, on its own is not enough to encourage long-term weight loss. The Academy of Nutrition and Dietetics recommends the best approach to long-term, sustained weight loss as a combination of both healthy diets and exercise.

A Quick Word of Advice

As with any other fasting method, exercise regime or change in your routine, it is always best to consult your doctor or health professional before embarking on a new process. A doctor who is already familiar with your medical history and background would be the best option in this instance because they will be able to advise you about what you need to be cautious of and how to take care of yourself during the fasting period. Talk to your health professional about what your goals are, why you're choosing to undergo this fasting method and about what to expect. At any point when you find yourself feeling unwell, you should stop and consult your health professional immediately.

Chapter 5: Water Fasting Mistakes to Avoid

Fasting has been practiced for thousands of years by people all over the world. Back then, it was done primarily for either spiritual or religious reasons. In modern times, it is reclaiming its popularity for a myriad of health reasons—with weight loss and improving overall bodily functions being a few of them.

Why fasting is such a great medium to achieving better, overall, and more importantly, prolonged good health is because it is one of the most powerful yet inexpensive tools that you have at your disposal. Everyone has access to it (as long as your doctor gives you the green light, of course). Who knew that by simply abstaining from food, you could achieve numerous benefits—including speeding up your weight loss goals, improving your mental clarity, enhancing the cell repairs happening within your body, lowering your blood pressure, and more?

While fasting can certainly be beneficial, those who are new to the practice tend to fall prey to one thing—*committing common fasting mistakes*. Mistakes prevent them from reaping the full benefits of their fasting sessions. Fasting may be good for you. However, when it feels too strenuous, difficult, and challenging, questions will start creeping into your mind—

dangerous questions like, *"Why am I doing this? Is this worth it?"*

With fasting mistakes, there are signs that you can look out for. The symptoms may not necessarily be the same since they vary from person to person. Fasting, once you've adapted to it, should improve your energy levels, mental clarity, and just healthier overall. Some quick signs that may indicate that you're experiencing signs of fasting mistakes include:

- Low energy levels (sometimes to the point of fatigue or being unable to function normally)
- Feeling a "mental fog," where you're finding it hard even to think straight sometimes
- Constant cravings that just won't seem to go away, which is often a sign of low blood sugar levels
- Dizziness, which can arise due to several causes, which include low blood sugar, a lack of salts in your body, perhaps even not being hydrated enough
- Frequent headaches
- Constipation

Common Water Fasting Mistakes to Stay Away From

While fasting can be great for your health, many people tend to give up along the way because they experience the frustration of not seeing the results they were hoping or expecting. What they don't realize is, they may have been making these common fasting mistakes, which inevitably led to the ineffectiveness of their regime. To save yourself from experience that same frustration, here are several basic water fasting mistakes that you should avoid:

Avoiding Sugary Drinks - This includes drinks which claim to be "calorie-free," like Diet Coke for example. Dr. Josh Axe, a certified doctor of natural medicine, highlighted in an article published on his website about just how unhealthy this supposed "diet" drinks can be. According to Dr. Axe, the artificial sweeteners which are contained in these drinks cause your body confusion, hindering its ability to manage hunger properly, and this (over time) leads to more weight gain. Those who consume far too many diet drinks are also twice as likely as anyone else to develop metabolic syndrome, according to Dr. Axe. Moreover, these diet drinks increase your chances of depression by as much as 30%. The point of a water fast is to give your body a chance to cleanse its system, to replenish in the healthiest possible way—which means you need to stay away from not only unhealthy foods but unhealthy drinks as well. Especially if one of your goals during this fast is to lose some weight. Any drinks which are not water will contain some amount of sugar in it, and sugar means calories. Water is the healthiest thing that you can put into your body, so embrace it and commit to it during your fast period.

Exercising Too Intensely During Your Fast - While it is okay to exercise when you're fasting, you need to be careful not to do too much. Another common mistake that often gets made is not adjusting your workout routine to match your fasted state. When you're fasting, your body has access to less food than what it normally would have, which means you could get tired much faster and doing intense routines is going to tire you quickly. On the days when you are fasting, you should aim to perform workouts which are lower in intensity, so you're not putting too much strain on your body and pushing yourself more than you should. It is best to consult your doctor before you do to ensure you're doing everything you can to take care of your health.

Doing Too Many Fast Days a Week - Understandably, you may be eager to jump right in (especially if you're new to this process) and try to get in as many fast days in a week as possible. The more you do, the better and quicker the results, right? Not necessarily. A common misconception is that more is better, just like exercising or eating nutritious food. However, fasting works a little differently. Experts recommend that you fast only 2 to 4 times a week, especially when you're first starting out. Why this range is recommended is because your body may start negatively reacting if you attempt to fast any more than this number. Your metabolism, everyday performance, and appetite are going to be greatly affected if your body "thinks" that it is going into starvation mode, which may happen when fasting is done far too frequently. Avoid the mistake of doing far too much too soon, as it's only going to be counter-productive to the positive benefits you want to achieve.

Giving Up Too Quickly - Fasting is certainly not easy, especially for beginners. Depriving yourself of your regular meals, staying away from food for a prolonged period, which is more than you're used to, and fighting the temptation not to give in when the smell of delicious food wafts your way—not to mention the strain on your body because it's running on fewer calories than what it may be accustomed to—all these lead to the fact that fasting requires discipline, mental toughness, willpower, and more to stay on course. When your body is going through the changes, you experience during the fast, and affecting you especially in the early stages, it can be tempting to throw in the towel and say that this isn't for you—but remind yourself about why you started this journey in the first place, and use that as the fuel and motivation that you need to keep going. Remember that it is always the hardest in the beginning, but it will get easier along the way.

Holding onto the Deprivation Mindset - It's a mind over matter situation when it comes to fasting. Yes, you are depriving your body, but *for a good reason.* You're doing this for your own good, and you need to focus on the positive and remind yourself that this is for your benefit. If you constantly hold onto the deprivation mindset, thinking about the food that you're missing out on, eventually your will power will only break down, and you'll give in to the urge to eat. It is important to focus on the positive because it is going to get you much further than a negative attitude ever will. It is all about perception and how you view things.

You're Far Too Stressed - Performing your fast when you're in a highly stressed out state can backfire on you. Stress increases your cortisol hormones, and because cortisol has a catabolic element to it, it is going to promote the breakdown of your body's tissues. When you're in a fasted state, your body is tapping into your fat stores to *preserve* the muscle tissue in your body, so higher levels of cortisol are going to be a problem.

Not Being Outdoors Enough - You do need to take it easy when you fast, but not *too easy*. You should still try to maintain as much of your regular routine as possible. Keeping an optimistic mindset and outlook. Staying indoors throughout the day and not moving about enough will only make you feel lethargic, and you'll find it harder to distract yourself from thinking about your fast. Constantly watching the clock wondering when it's going to be over is not the way to go, because it won't be long before you eventually give up since the effort will not feel worth your time. Go for a walk, get some fresh air, go for a light jog around the park, anything to get up and get moving. Remember to stay hydrated throughout your movements though. Even when you're at work, get up, walk around, take active work breaks to help clear your mind. Walk around the office, smile and greet your co-workers and your day will seem so much better. The less you think about your fast, the quicker the time will pass. Even better, you'll be more inclined to stick to the regime long term when you see how easy it is to get through the day after all.

Chapter 6: Water Fasting FAQs and Goal-Setting

You're about to embark on a journey that's about to change your health for the better (if done correctly). Any kind of change can be nerve-wracking and maybe even a little bit frightening at times because this is not something we're accustomed to. Any time we need to get pushed out of our comfort zone, it will be a challenging affair. Beginning a fasting ritual is no different.

Frequently Asked Questions (FAQs) About Water Fasting

As with anything new that you've never done before, questions are bound to be on your mind. Whether you're a beginner or seasoned water faster, there may be a couple of questions you may have about this process or about fasting, in general.

Q: Is there a difference between starving and fasting since both involve abstaining from food?

A: Yes, there is. Fasting is something that is done intentionally and with purpose. You're doing it for health reasons, and you're *choosing* to undergo this process for the benefits that you're hoping to get out it. Starving, on the other hand, sometimes cannot be helped. There aren't any benefits that are going to come with starvation because it is an unplanned process.

Q: Is there a reason why I shouldn't be fasting?

A: Yes, under several circumstances, you should not be undergoing a fast as it might serve to affect your health negatively. Fasting is supposed to be beneficial, but that is assuming that you're completely fit and healthy when you're performing the fast. There are certain circumstances where fasting may not be the best approach to take. These include if you're under the age of 18 for example, if you're not feeling well, pregnant, undergoing specific medication for pre-existing health conditions, nursing or suffering from any ailments which may be made worse through fasting. It is always best to consult with your doctor before undergoing any change in your routine that is going to affect you physically.

Q: I'm already healthy, why the need to fast?

A: The same reason why we take showers, brush our teeth, and comb our hair every morning. We're already clean, but we do it routinely every day, anyway, as it makes us look and feel good. Well, fasting is the same—but this time, instead of focusing on the external, you're now focusing on the *internal* part of your body. Water fasting is the healthiest way for you to cleanse and detox your body from within, which in the long run will keep your internal organs working well for a long time. It may not feel good depriving yourself of the delicious food you're so tempted to it, but your body will thank you for it in the long run.

Q: Am I really allowed to ONLY have water during a water fast?

A: Ideally, water should be your best friend. After all, it is water fast. However, if you're looking to make the experience a little more pleasurable, there are other beverage forms which you could consume. What you **shouldn't** consume is sugary, soda drinks, diet drinks or any other zero-calorie drinks which claim to have "no sugar" in them. What you can consume, however, if you *really* feel like you need a pick me up, is tea, lime juice, perhaps even an apple cider vinegar mix. Minimizing your sugar intake is the key because the whole point of this fast is that it is supposed to reset your body from all the unhealthy junk that usually goes into it.

Q: Will fasting make me look any different?

A: Well, there may be no *significant* visible difference immediately, but you will feel better after doing it for a certain time. The physical difference may only come in much later. Perhaps when you've lost some weight, or your skin has cleared up and looking more radiant and younger because of the extra hydration you're getting from all that extra water intake.

Q: What can I expect during my water fast?

A: You can expect it to be challenging in the beginning, especially if this is something that you have never done before. During your fast, you'll feel significantly less bloated, although you may struggle with hunger pangs, which may affect you a lot when you're new to the process. You may experience other symptoms, including fatigue and mild headaches. Not everyone is going to experience the same symptoms, as some people take to fasting much better than others. You'll also learn to appreciate food much more when you get to eat again since nothing makes you appreciate what you have more than not being able to *have it when you want it.*

Q: What if I were just to cut calories instead of doing a full on water fast? Won't it have the same benefits?

A: No, it will not. Restricting your body of the calories that it needs will only serve to slow your metabolism down. This, in turn, will make you feel foggy, lethargic and constantly hungry, craving more food which may lead to binging when you eventually don't have the willpower to resist the urge to eat anymore. Your body slows down its metabolism because it is trying to match the limited calories that it is now being fed. Fasting, on the other hand, won't slow down your metabolism because there's no calorie intake coming in for it to match, and therefore, your metabolism now does the *opposite.* Your growth hormone gets stimulated; your adrenaline levels are higher; you feel that your body kicks it into high gear. Do you notice how you tend to feel sleepy or groggy when you've eaten far too much, especially after lunch? Well, without food coming into your digestive system during the day, there's more blood flow heading to your brain now to keep it feeling sharp and alert. You won't feel hungry all the time either—the hunger pangs will come and go during the day, especially when you're not thinking about it all the time.

Setting Goals to Ensure Success

Fasting is not going to be like anything you have done before. It process, more than any other, is going to be a battle of willpower. It's going to be mind over matter—which is why it's important to set goals for this process too, as with any other important undertaking in your life.

Goals help you set realistic expectations, and give you something to work for. It serves as a reminder as to why you're doing this, gives you a mission and a purpose. The act of setting goals is going to be just the motivation that you need to keep going at the points where you feel like giving up the most. You started this process with a goal - or several goals - in mind. There's a *reason why* you did this. What you need now is further motivation to keep moving one more step forward.

If you're about to embark on your water fasting journey - *whether for the first time or if you're looking for a motivation to keep pushing forward* - here are some motivating reminders to help you better stick to your goals:

Manage Your Expectations - Especially if your goal is to lose weight. There are no shortcuts to losing weight, as much as we wished that there was. Fasting can help, but that's not its primary purpose. Fasting is for overall better health, and this is what you need to remind yourself of when setting goals. Expecting miraculous results is only going to lead to disappointment, which will only make you want to give up. Try making your goal about health instead of focusing too much on weight loss.

Take It One Day At a Time - You've probably heard this advice about taking baby steps so often that you're thinking, *"Oh, this again."* However, there's a reason this is constantly touted as a step that you should take when you're working on achieving your goal. Trying to do too much too soon has never proven to be a long term effective method, but taking baby steps and taking it one day at a time makes coping with the process so much easier.

Writing Down Your Purpose - Sometimes, you just need to see that physical remind in front of you to remind yourself about what you're doing and why you're doing it. Mentally reminding yourself works too, but having a physical reminder in front of you - whether it is on a post-it note, on your mobile or desktop wallpaper, or even written down in your notebook - is going to work even better. Humans are very visual creatures, and we sometimes need to see things in front of us to believe in it. Goal reminders work in pretty much the same way.

Be Committed - Because you owe it to yourself to do this for your health. You only have one body, and we often take health for granted until there comes a day when we wish we could go back to being healthy again. Don't wait until the moment comes—instead, be committed to taking care of the body that you have right now. Exercise, eat right, fast, and do what you need to do to keep your body healthy for as long as you possibly can. Your future self with thank you for it down the road.

Chapter 7: Fasting Made Easy (or Easier)

Revered by the ancients as one of the most effective forms of healing the body, fasting is reclaiming its popularity as society starts to take health seriously once more. Despite its tremendous benefits, not everyone is going to find fasting an easy process. There will be times where it is going to challenge you and push your willpower to its very end—but if you can persevere and stick it out, you will emerge triumphant at the end of this process.

Luckily, there are a few strategies and practical tips available to help your body adjust and get more comfortable with the fasting process—even giving you the ability to go on for longer fasting periods once you've done this several times. Think of fasting like a non-physical form of exercise. Exercising is hard in the beginning, isn't it? However, once you've built that momentum, it starts to get easier—perhaps even enjoyable. Water fasting is going to be in the same process. It's going to be hard, maybe even weird in the beginning because we're so used to consuming regular meals, but eventually, it gets easier.

Preparing Your Body — Strategies to Help Make the Water Fasting Process Easier

A water fast is going to be a shock to the system for some. Imagine not being able to consume anything but water for several hours during the day. That's going to be a challenge, and you're going to need the following tips to ease yourself into it:

Creating a Schedule for Yourself - Things always seem more manageable when there's an organized system in place. It works with water fasting too. When creating your fasting schedule, think about creating one that is low in stress. One of the reasons that many people fall off the wagon and don't see their fasting through is due to high levels of stress since it doesn't do your body any favors. It is highly recommended that you plan out your fasting schedule on the days which are going to be less stressful for you. If you have a high powered, high stress job, perhaps think about doing the fast during the weekends when you've got some downtime. A schedule which is low in stress is going to be especially crucial during the first few fasts sessions because this is where you need to stick it out the most.

Stay Away from Negative People - There are many reasons to stay away from negative people—and now, water fast is one of them. Sometimes, it may seem impossible because these negative individuals could be your friends, family, or co-workers, which just makes avoiding them, well, unavoidable. If this is the case, you might have to think about sitting down with them and having a serious discussion. Gently explain to them what you plan to do, and let them know you would appreciate their support and encouragement during this process. Positive reinforcement is crucial for the success of your water fast process because negativity is only going to make you want to give up and throw in the towel even more.

Have Salts on Hand - Your insulin levels are going to take a dip during your fast, and because of that, your body is going to retain its sodium. Insulin is responsible for the sugar that is within your cells, and when there's a drop in your insulin levels, the body starts retaining its sodium. This explains why some people may experience dizziness, perhaps even tiredness during the fast. If this is what you're experiencing, a pinch of salt on your tongue with a glass of water is going to help you significantly.

Pleasure Day - Everyone needs a little reward to keep them going. Fasting is hard work, and you should reward yourself for sticking through the process. Every fast day that you overcome is one step closer towards your goal of better health. Take a day off to reward yourself. A good spa day, for example, can do wonders to elevate your mood and relieve your stress, and if you opt for a spa day *on the same day* as your water fast, it'll just make the entire process a lot more enjoyable. If a spa day is not your forte, consider another (lightweight) activity that puts you in a good mood. Something that you look forward to.

Stay Out of the Kitchen - This goes without saying. If you want to avoid temptation, you need to stay away from where the temptation is. Food cravings and temptation is going to be one of your biggest struggles during the water fast, so until you get used to the process, try to avoid the kitchen as much as possible on the days that you're doing your fast. Get rid of all the junk food in your pantry too so that you won't be tempted to undergo binge eating once your fast is over.

Think About Strategic Drinking - Hunger pangs tend to strike during the times when you're accustomed to having your regular meals. That's perfectly normal, because of the hunger hormone- ghrelin - which is kicking in. This is where planning to drink strategically is going to help. During the times that you know you're going to feel hungry the most, plan to consume a lot of water during this time. A nice herbal or chamomile tea would also be helpful. Remember, no soda or carbonated drinks.

It's Okay to Get Some Rest - If you need a little time out for a few minutes during your fast day, give yourself permission to do so. This is easier when your fast is done during the weekends since you'll have more flexibility in your schedule. At work, a quick water break or 5-minute walk around to give yourself a break would help. You may feel the urge to rest when you're just starting out on your fast since your body is adjusting to the new changes which it is going through.

Mentally Prepare Yourself for the Process - The idea of fasting, especially if you're doing it for multiple days, can be a daunting thing to think about. Mental preparation is just as necessary as physical preparation. You've got to be prepared for what's in store. Read motivational books, talk to others who have done the water fast before, get friends on board for emotional support. Perhaps even watch motivational or educational videos about people who have gone through fasts before. Get on board with the *Yes! I can do it!!* Attitude. The winning attitude.

Think About Transitioning into the Process - If jumping right in with both feet is not the best approach for you, take a step back and think about transitioning into the process. Start easing yourself into the process by cutting out sugar drinks first and then slowly weaning yourself off processed foods. Reduce the portion size that you eat during your regular meals. Do this for at least 2 or 3 days leading up to your fast, and this will make the water fasting process a lot easier.

Long Haul Fasts Should Be Done Under Supervision - Fasting for a long period can take a toll on your body, especially if you're doing it for more than 3-days. If you're attempting this, do it with the supervised help of a trained professional who can monitor your situation and guide you whenever necessary. A trained expert who has dealt with many clients who have undergone the water fast before would be your best bet. Ask around, do your research, or even ask your usual health practitioner if they know of anyone they can recommend.

Getting Plenty of Sleep - On average, we need about 7 to 8 hours of sleep in a day for good health. An even more reason to get in this recommended hours of sleep when you're undergoing water fast is that you're likely to experience a drop in your energy levels, perhaps even stamina if you're doing this for more than a day. Maintaining a healthy sleep pattern is a must, or you're going to find yourself struggling significantly from a lack of food and a lack of energy to add to that. As much as you would like to push yourself, don't. *Now* is when you need to listen to your body—more than ever.

Track Your Progress - This lets you see just how far you've come, and how much closer you are to your goals. With you trying to progress forward without any sustainable way of measuring, it won't be long before you start to wonder whether you're making any progress or not. That's because you won't be able to clearly see how far you've come, how many steps forward you've already taken from where you first started out.

When you feel like you're not making any progress, the temptation to give up will get stronger over time. That is why you need a good system for tracking your progress throughout this water fasting journey. Keep a journal that documents where you first started on day one, and continue all throughout. Whenever you feel like you could use some motivation, or a reminder to keep moving forward, reflect back to your progress from day one and see just how far you've come.

Conclusion

In Review

Potential Benefits of Water Fasting

Water fasting has been linked with a variety of health benefits in human and animal studies.

Here are a few health benefits of water fasting.

It May Promote Autophagy

Autophagy is a process where old parts of your cells are broken down and recycled.

Several studies have found that autophagy may help protect against diseases like cancer, Alzheimer's disease and heart disease.

For example, autophagy may prevent damaged parts of your cells from accumulating, which is a risk factor for many cancers. This may help prevent cancer cells from growing.

Research from animal studies consistently finds that water fasting helps promote autophagy. Animal studies also show that autophagy may help extend lifespan.

That said, there are very few human studies on water fasting, autophagy and disease prevention. More research is needed before recommending it to promote autophagy.

It May Help Lower Blood Pressure

Research shows that longer, medically supervised water fasts may help people with high blood pressure lower their blood pressure.

In one study, 68 people who had borderline high blood pressure, water fasted for nearly 14 days under medical supervision.

At the end of the fast, 82% of people saw their blood pressure fall to healthy levels (120/80 mmHg). Additionally, the average drop in blood pressure was 20 mmHg for systolic (upper value) and 7 mmHg for diastolic (lower value), which is significant.

In another study, 174 people with high blood pressure water fasted for an average of 10 to 11 days.

At the end of the fast, 90% of people achieved a blood pressure lower than 140/90 mmHg — the limits used to diagnose high blood pressure. Additionally, the average fall in systolic blood pressure (upper value) was a substantial 37 mmHG .

Unfortunately, there are no human studies that investigate the link between short-term water fasts (24 to 72 hours) and blood pressure.

It May Improve Insulin and Leptin Sensitivity

Insulin and leptin are important hormones that affect the body's metabolism. Insulin helps the body store nutrients from the bloodstream, while leptin helps the body feel full.

Research shows that water fasting could make your body more sensitive to leptin and insulin. Greater sensitivity makes these hormones more effective.

For example, being more insulin sensitive means your body is more efficient at reducing blood sugar. Meanwhile, being more leptin sensitive could help your body process hunger signals more efficiently and, in turn, may lower your risk of obesity.

It May Lower the Risk of Several Chronic Diseases

There is some evidence that water fasting may lower the risk of chronic diseases like diabetes, cancer and heart disease.

In one study, 30 healthy adults followed a water fast for 24 hours. After the fast, they had significantly lower blood levels of cholesterol and triglycerides — two risk factors for heart disease.

Several animal studies have also found that water fasting may protect the heart against damage from free radicals.

Free radicals are unstable molecules that can damage parts of cells. They are known to play a role in many chronic diseases.

Moreover, research on animals has found that water fasting may suppress genes that help cancer cells grow. It may also improve the effects of chemotherapy.

Keep in mind, there are only a handful of studies that look at the impact of water fasting in humans. More research on humans is needed before making recommendations.

Your chosen length of time for fasting must always be the right length for you at the time you are considering it. Remember always to listen to your body at every stage of the process and never to push yourself too far. Take it one step at a time and one day at a time. You'll eventually get to your goals without having to do too much and too soon. Fasting is supposed to be beneficial for your body and to improve your overall health—hence, stay safe throughout your process, and you'll be reaping the benefits that you hoped for and more in no time.

Finally, if you found this book useful in anyway, a review on Amazon is always appreciated!

Summary Notes

What happens to your body during a fast?

Is fasting safe, or is it simply another quick way to lose weight?

What *is water fasting*, anyway?

Water Fasting: Lose Your Weight Fast, Cleanse Your Body, and Revitalize Your Health Through Water Fasting is a comprehensive guide that will aid you through the following areas:

- A look at the history of fasting and its effects on the human body;
- The stages of water fasting that you need to go through;
- How to perform water fasting;
- What water fasting mistakes you should avoid;
- Common FAQs about water fasting answered;
- How to set goals to keep you moving forward; and
- Easy-to-follow strategies that will help make your water fasting process easier on your body.

Understanding the science of water fasting is crucial to doing it right. You do not want to go about doing a fast without knowing the how-to's and even the why's. Fasting is beneficial for your health—but *only if* it is performed in the right way.

If you're ready, let your water fasting journey begin!

References

- https://www.healthline.com/nutrition/water-fasting#section6

- https://www.allaboutfasting.com/master-cleanse.html

- https://www.allaboutfasting.com/benefits-of-fasting.html

- https://www.healthline.com/nutrition/how-to-fast#section9

- https://drjockers.com/water-fasting/

- https://www.ncbi.nlm.nih.gov/pubmed/12470446

- https://www.ncbi.nlm.nih.gov/pubmed/11416824

- https://www.ncbi.nlm.nih.gov/pubmed/16299415

- https://www.ncbi.nlm.nih.gov/pmc/articles/PMC156352/

- https://www.ncbi.nlm.nih.gov/pmc/articles/PMC3946160/

- https://www.globalhealingcenter.com/natural-health/health-benefits-of-water-fasting/

- https://www.medicalnewstoday.com/articles/319835.php

- https://wellnessmama.com/345549/water-fasting/

- https://www.livestrong.com/article/70706-rapid-weight-loss-water-fasting/

- https://www.everydayhealth.com/water-health/water-body-health.aspx

- https://www.everydayhealth.com/water-health/water-body-health.aspx

- https://www.fastingblog.com/water-fasting-pros-and-cons/

- https://medium.com/@jeromehuff/you-need-to-avoid-these-5-mistakes-when-you-fast-ba7573ab14b3

- https://www.natural-health-zone.com/water-fasting.html

- https://www.wikihow.com/Perform-a-Water-Fast

- https://www.globalhealingcenter.com/natural-health/stages-of-fasting-what-happens-when-you-fast/

- https://drjockers.com/water-fasting/

- https://www.wikihow.com/Prepare-for-Fasting

- https://observer.com/2017/06/most-common-intermittent-fasting-mistakes/

- https://whatsgood.vitaminshoppe.com/intermittent-fasting-mistakes/

- https://theunconventionalroute.com/water-fasting-tips/

- https://www.dummies.com/health/nutrition/weight-loss/set-realistic-expectations-and-goals-for-fasting/

- https://www.success.com/9-ways-to-achieve-your-biggest-goals-quickly/

- https://www.huffingtonpost.com/bradley-foster/how-to-set-goals_b_3226083.html

- https://drjockers.com/water-fasting/

- https://www.wikihow.com/Perform-a-Water-Fast

- https://www.inc.com/susan-steinbrecher/10-quick-tips-to-help-you-stick-to-your-goals.html

www.ingramcontent.com/pod-product-compliance
Lightning Source LLC
Chambersburg PA
CBHW072112280526
45788CB00006B/2501